TOMATO

LYCOPENE

POWER!

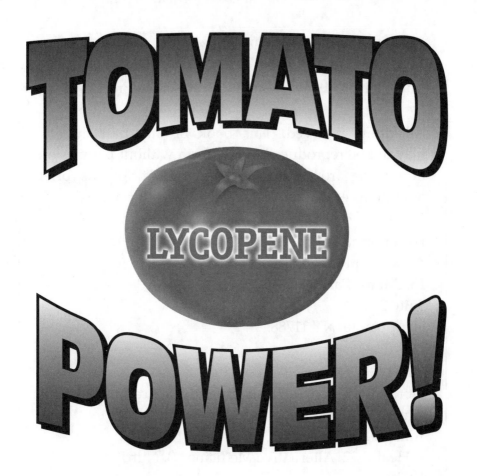

TOMATO

LYCOPENE

POWER!

The Miracle Nutrient That Can Prevent
Aging, Heart Disease and Cancer

by James F. Scheer

Forward by

JAMES F. BALCH, MD

Co-author of Prescription for Nutritional Healing

For information contact:
Advanced Research Press
150 Motor Parkway
Suite 210
Hauppauge, NY 11788

FIRST EDITION
Library of Congress Cataloging-in-Publication Data
James F. Scheer
Tomato Power
1. Health   2. Alternative Medicine   3. Nutrition
1. Title
ISBN 1-889462-04-7

Printed in the United States of America

Published by: Advanced Research Press,Inc.
                       150 Motor Parkway
                       Suite 210
                       Hauppauge, NY 11788

Publisher/President: Steve Blechman

Managing Director: Roy Ulin

Art Director: Rob Wilner (DotCom)

Copy Editor: Carol Goldberg

Cover Design: Sam Powell

Printed by: DotCom

DEDICATION

This book is dedicated to scientists and researchers throughout the world who have so diligently worked toward the discovery, quantification and documentation of the amazing health benefits and protective powers of lycopene, a true super-antioxidant. As a result of their fine efforts, millions of people will be able to enjoy better health and longer productive lives.

The material presented in this book is for informational purposes only. It is not intended to serve as a prescription for you, or to replace the advice of your medical professional. Consult your physician before beginning any new conventional or alternative therapy suggested herein. If you have any medical conditions or are taking any prescription or non-prescription medications, consult your medical professional before beginning any new therapy or discontinuing the medications or treatments that your are currently using. The author and the publisher disclaim any liability or loss, personal and otherwise, resulting from the advice in this book. The material presented herein is not a substitute for the advice of a personal health care professional. Use of the information herein is at the risk solely of the reader.

TABLE OF CONTENTS

About the Forward Author

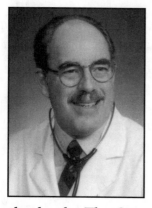

James F. Balch

A urologist and certified nutritional consultant, Dr. James F. Balch also holds a Master's degree in theology and urban ministry. He has co-authored two best-selling books, *Prescription for Nutritional Healing* and *Prescription for Dietary Wellness*, and is the author of the book, *The Super Anti-Oxidants* and of the widely respected newsletter, *Prescription for Healthy Living*. Convinced there was a better way to achieve good health than to "take two aspirin and call me in the morning," Dr. Balch has devoted the past 15 of his 30 years in medicine to a worldwide search for more effective ways to treat and cure disease. He lectures extensively in the United States and Canada, exhorting audiences in person and on radio and television to free themselves from the shackles of a narrow-minded pharmaceutical-based health care delivery system by assuming an active role in maintaining their own good health.

ABOUT THE AUTHOR

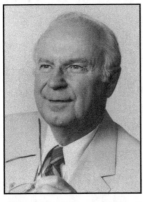

James F. Scheer

Editor of three health/nutrition magazines — *Food-Wise, Health Freedom News* and *Let's Live* — James F. Scheer has also authored 20 books and contributed thousands of articles to leading publications in the United States, Canada and England, including: *Cosmopolitan, Esquire, Good Housekeeping, Redbook* and *Science Digest. Solved: The Riddle of Illness,* a perennial best-seller written with Stephen Langer, M.D., is one of the first books to reveal an often undetected medical condition -- low thyroid function that saps energy and leads to sexual disorders and diminished ability to think and remember. His latest effort with Dr. Langer, entitled *Raise Your IQ Sky High!,* discusses how nutrients, hormones and certain exercises can upgrade thinking and remembering.

Recipient of the 1978 Caveat Emptor Award from Caveat Emptor magazine for his contributions to educating American consumers in health and nutrition, Scheer was one of the first writers to popularize use of the trace mineral selenium after conducting in-depth research into relevant literature and finding that, taken in judicious amounts, it is a powerful anti-cancer nutrient. He also coined the term "secondhand smoke" to describe the effects of cigarette smoke in the environment. In a new project, he is writing a book introducing chia seed – a food noted among pre-Columbian civilizations for its strength and energy-giving properties – to the American public.

"Dangerously one-sided psychology textbooks ignore nutrition as relevant to emotional and mental health," says Scheer.

FORWARD

First, I would like to congratulate you for reading this book. You are taking an active role in your own health management. This is a good thing. It will change not only your health, but your entire life. You have respect for your own body, and it will lead you to a more healthy, prosperous life.

One of the most important things you must understand to begin truly managing your health is the oxygen paradox. Although as humans we need oxygen to live, the byproducts of oxygen metabolism cause free radical damage that prematurely ages the body. This oxygen paradox has only begun to be understood in the last 20 years. Oxidative stress is easy to see if you cut open an apple. It begins to rot almost immediately due to exposure to oxygen. This same rotting is occurring in our bodies all the time. But there is something you can do to combat this oxidative stress. When antioxidants are present in the body, they dramatically reduce the damage caused by oxidative stress.

Free radical damage and oxidative stress are linked to both cancer and heart disease, the two major killers in the U.S. and Canada, as well as many other degenerative diseases. As an antioxidant, lycopene, a carotenoid, has a remarkable preventative effect on prostate cancer as well as other cancers, and it has changed my impression of this disease. Additionally, lycopene helps prevent the growth of breast, lung, gastrointestinal, cervical and endometrial cancer cells. There is more lycopene found in the human body than any other of the carotenoids (including beta-carotene), and its highest concentrations are found in the testes, prostate, adrenal gland, ovaries, liver and lungs.

The most common food source for lycopene is tomato sauce and ketchup. It seems to offer the best absorption when combined and cooked with oils.

As a physician and urologist who has treated many prostate cancer victims, I know there are few options outside of radical surgery, hormone manipulation and radiation to effect a cure for prostate cancer. There are currently no medicines available that will prevent this horrifying disease which kills 50,000 men each year. Lycopene has definitely changed my understanding of prostate cancer, and how one should approach its prevention and probably its treatment. As lycopene is studied more extensively, it will change the way we treat cancer in the 21st century.

Lycopene also defends the body against other lethal diseases like arteriosclerosis. A leader in the study of lipid metabolism, Dr. Michael Aviram, of Rambam Medical Center in Haifa, Israel, shared with me the importance of antioxidants, particularly lycopene, in preventing the beginnings of arteriosclerosis. LDL cholesterol becomes harmful, sticking to the walls of the arteries, when it is oxidized. In their laboratory, Dr. Aviram and his associates have demonstrated that Lyc-O-Mato, an all natural tomato lycopene supplement, has been shown to prevent the formation of the arteriosclerotic plaque and stop the progression of the plaque buildup. In a significant percentage of the animals tested that had advanced arteriosclerosis, the Lyc-O-Mato was actually able to turn the process around, decreasing plaque buildup.

Based on these findings, I believe that blood antioxidant levels should be tested just like cholesterol levels so people can supplement their deficiencies. More of these antioxidant blood tests are becoming available. They're not easy to find, but physicians are beginning to use them as a testing point to determine the overall oxidative stress in the body.

I was privileged to learn firsthand of the work being done to produce all natural lycopene supplements. A company called LycoRed has done extensive work in Israel to create a pure lycopene extract (Lyc-O-Mato) that allows scientists to research lycopene extensively through the use of lycopene supplements. It was a breakthrough in the scientific investigation of lycopene. Until this point, synthetic supplements did not fit the requirements needed in experimental models in the laboratory. Dr. Zohar Nir is the visionary who saw the great potential of creating an all-natural tomato lycopene supplement.

I traveled to Israel and was escorted through LycoRed's special tomato patch. There I saw a remarkable difference between the super, lycopene-rich tomatoes they grow there and regular tomatoes you buy in U.S. supermarkets. These are not genetically engineered fruits, they are normal, hybridized tomatoes. It's quite apparent when you observe them that these tomatoes are different. They are a much deeper red than the average tomato, and are much fuller when cut open. I also saw how lycopene is extracted from these super tomatoes without chemicals to create all-natural tomato lycopene supplements.

We are entering a new era in health care, a real health revolution, where patients take an active role in managing their health. In my opinion, doctors will have to change their old ideas about health care, incorporating an integrated, complimentary approach in managing the diseases of the next millennium. I firmly believe this change will push natural substances to the forefront of health care, and lycopene is one of these important natural products.

James E. Balch, MD
Author of *The Super-Anti Oxidants*
Co-Author of *Prescription For Nutritional Healing*

Chapter 1
Lycopene: One of the Most Important Carotenoids

In this Age of Superlatives, high-thrust adjectives such as "stupendous," "terrific," and "incredible" are often lavished on ordinary things.

That's why it's refreshing to know about lycopene, an extraordinary nutrition-health product that actually deserves them. Lycopene is the little-known cousin of the well-known carotenoid, beta carotene, and is about to become much more well known.

A powerful nutrient in ripe red tomatoes, lycopene was recently spotlighted in a study by Edward Giovannucci, M.D., of the prestigious Harvard University School of Public Health. Dr. Giovannucci announced a remarkable health benefit in eating tomatoes, tomato sauce, ketchup and tomato paste-topped pizza more than twice weekly: *a 21 to 43 percent reduced risk of prostate cancer.*[1]

This was an important breakthrough for two reasons. First, prostate cancer is the most common cancer in U.S. males, causing between 40,000 and 50,000 deaths annually.

Increase in prostatic cancer incidence in the western world

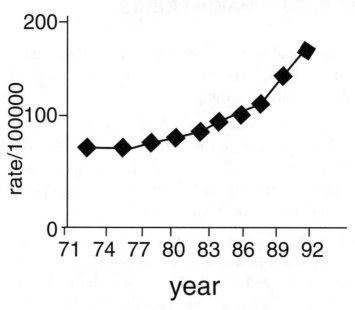

Prostatic cancer

Adapted from Mettlin C. Eur.J. Cancer 33, 340 - 1997

Second, research attention was directed away from beta carotene, then considered the most likely carotenoid to be able to prevent prostate cancer.

Dr. Giovannucci states that there is little evidence to support a prostate cancer benefit from fruits and vegetables. "Nevertheless, because of the great importance of this disease, we explored carotenoids in prostate cancer on our Health Professional Follow-Up Study."[2]

Trends in age-adjusted prostate cancer incidence and mortality rate per 100,000 in black and caucasion men in the United States 1973-1992 from the NGI Surveillance, Epidemiology, and End Results Program of the National Cancer Institute

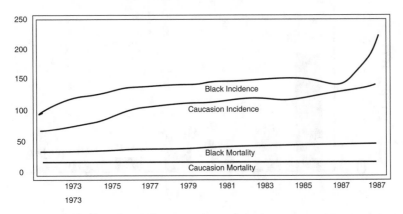

Adapted from European Journal of Cancer, Vol. 33 No. 3. pages 340-347, 1997

Research by Steven Clinton, Ph.D., of the Dana Farber Cancer Institute, gave more focus to this exploration. In examining cancerous prostate tissue, Dr. Clinton found that lycopene was the most plentiful carotenoid there.[3]

Concentration of lycopene in human tissues

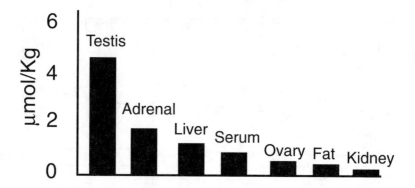

Adapted from: Stahl et al. Arch. Biochem. Biophys. 294, 173 - 1992

During a six year period, Dr. Giovannucci and his research team followed 800 cases of prostate cancer to see if there is a relationship between this form of cancer and the patients' intake of alpha carotene, beta carotene, beta-cryptoxanthin, lutein and lycopene.

A LITTLE FAT HELPS

The only nutrient that turned out to have significant preventive value was lycopene, wrote Dr. Giovannucci. He and associates also found that lycopene was most efficiently absorbed when accompanied by lipids (fats) in the diet.[4]

"Cooking tomatoes in oil encourages intestinal absorption and results in a two-to-threefold rise in plasma lycopene concentrations," states Dr. Giovannucci. "Tomato sauce is one of the best lycopene sources."

Proof of the tomato product's benefit is revealed in statistics showing that men from Mediterranean countries who eat a lot of tomatoes have lower rates of prostate cancer, whereas those in countries where tomato-eating is less common have higher rates.

Lycopene serum levels in various countries

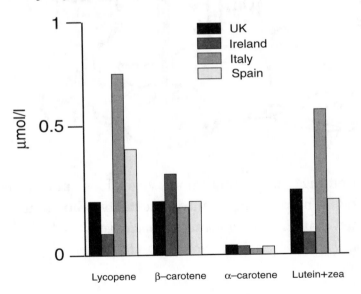

Lycopene: Important Carotenoid

There was a far lower incidence of prostate cancer in people eating the Mediterranean diet than in those eating African-American or Asian-American diets. The latter two groups customarily eat fewer tomato-based foods. Most remarkable is the fact that *even a family history of prostate cancer did not reduce lycopene's protective effect.*

Giovannucci urged men concerned about the possibility of prostate cancer to eat more "spaghetti smothered in tomato sauce."

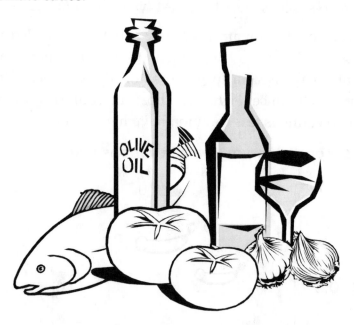

Admitting that eating more vegetables and fruits can often help reduce cancer mortality, Giovannucci claimed that *"it's the lycopene in tomato-based foods that is responsible for lowering the risk of prostate cancer."*

Protective benefits increase with an increased intake of tomato products, says Dr. Giovannucci, claiming that men who ate two or more servings a week averaged a 35 percent reduction in prostate cancer risk.

Effect of various tomato food products in relation to prostate cancer risk

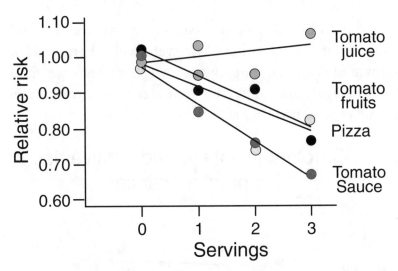

Adapted from Giovanucci et al. J. of National Cancer Inst. 87, 1767 - 1995

Relative to lycopene's possible benefits in a person already diagnosed with prostate cancer, Dr. Giovannucci writes that his team's findings don't rule out an effect of slowing such cancer development.

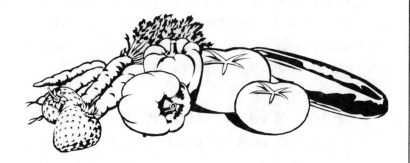

Some forms of prostate cancer are aggressive and highly fatal and others are relatively benign. Dr. Giovannucci noted that *tomato products are more beneficial in more aggressive cancers -- even those that have already spread to other parts of the body.*

Carotenoid intake and relative risk of prostate cancer

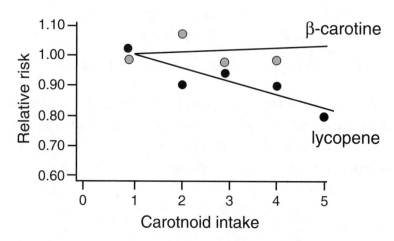

Adapted from Giovanucci et al. J. of National Cancer Inst. 87, 1767 - 1995

Studies by biochemists in the United States and Italy validated the Giovannucci findings. Distinguished researchers worldwide began discovering astonishing results from using lycopene in the prevention of various disorders, various kinds of cancer (in addition to prostate), cardiovascular conditions and other major diseases.

It strikes many people as strange that something so seemingly ordinary as the red substance taken from tomatoes can achieve such extraordinary results. Naturally, this makes them want to know more about lycopene, and there is much more to know.

Before getting into the lycopene story -- and it is a fascinating one -- it would be best to mention lycopene's family, the carotenoids. Carotenoids are the red, orange, and yellow coloring substances in plants and animals. They got their name from carrots, from which they were first derived.

Although beta is the second letter of the Greek alphabet, beta carotene was the first carotenoid isolated. Back in 1928, a chemist named B. von Euler made the significant discovery that it was the precursor of the body's most usable form of vitamin A.[5]

A molecule of beta carotene contains two units of pre-vitamin A, which the small intestine and the liver split into two molecules of vitamin A by means of an enzyme called beta carotene-15, 15' dioxygenase.

β-carotene

Empirical Formula : $CH_{40}H_{56}$
Molecular Weight : 536.85

Remember from high school chemistry that an enzyme is a compound that causes a reaction without being involved in that reaction?

Some people take for granted that beta carotene automatically converts into vitamin A. This is not so. If there's too little of this specific enzyme, the translation can't take place. Also, diabetics and people with low thyroid function have difficulty bringing about this conversion.

lycopene

Empirical Formula : $CH_{40}H_{56}$
Molecular Weight : 536.85

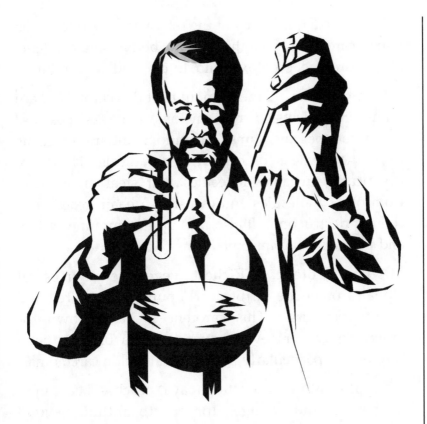

Of the 600 discovered carotenoids -- most of them not as yet sufficiently studied -- beta carotene appears to be the only one capable of producing two molecules of vitamin A. Some carotenoids can produce one molecule of vitamin A. Others are not chemically structured to permit conversion into vitamin A. Lycopene is one of the latter.

Let's take a quick look at the relatives of lycopene, the major carotenoids in the human body: beta-carotene, alpha-carotene, cryptoxanthin, lutein, and zeaxanthin.

Beta-carotene. Largest amounts of this carotenoid are found in apricots, carrots, melons, papayas, peaches, sweet potatoes and yams. An antioxidant, it protects us from the ravages of certain free radicals. These are chemically unstable molecules that steal an electron from other molecules and can start a chain reaction of cellular destruction. It also revs up the immune system and protects us from some forms of cancer.

Alpha-carotene. Richest vegetable sources of alpha-carotene are carrots, corn, pumpkin, and red and yellow peppers. This carotene is best known for inhibiting cancers even better than its brother, beta-carotene — particularly lung, liver and skin carcinomas.

Cryptoxanthin. Look to papaya, peaches, nectarines, tangerines and oranges for cryptoxanthin. Several studies show that a high intake of this carotenoid reduces the risk of cervical cancer.

Lutein. Some of the less popular vegetables boast liberal amounts of lutein: broccoli, collard greens, kale, mustard greens and spinach. A strong antioxidant, lutein is thought to team up with zeaxanthin to protect against ailments of the retina of the eye, particularly macular degeneration. Several well-structured studies show that these carotenoids are indeed strongly represented in the eyes. However, they indicate that lycopene is the best carotenoid protector against macular degeneration. Please see the Beaver Dam study discussed later in this book.

Zeaxanthin. Like its close relative, lutein, zeaxanthin can be found mainly in broccoli, collard greens, kale, mustard greens and spinach, but also in beet greens, chicory, cress leaf, okra and Swiss chard. It is also richly present in the macula of the eyes and thought to be biological insurance against macular degeneration. Like lutein, it seems to be garnering credit that should go to lycopene. A powerful antioxidant, zeaxanthin protects against peroxide free radicals and guards sensitive cell membranes against damage.

Various studies show that lycopene makes up at least 50 percent of the carotenoids in the human body, accentuating its importance. Although tomatoes are the best source of lycopene, by far, it can also be found in watermelon, pink grapefruit and apricots in small amounts.

If you eat a ripe red tomato, will you absorb large amounts of lycopene?

Not necessarily, unless you take in some fat along with it. Lycopene authority John W. Erdman, Jr. and associates tell us that no lycopene from tomato juice appears in your blood plasma unless that juice was heated first.[6]

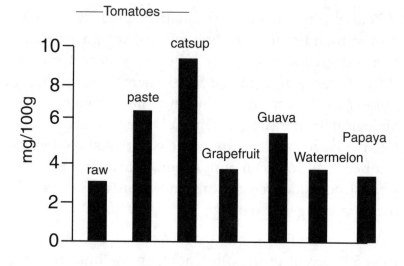

Lycopene content of foods

——Tomatoes——

mg/100g

- catsup
- paste
- raw
- Grapefruit
- Guava
- Watermelon
- Papaya

adapted from: Gerster H.J. Amer.Coll. Nut. 16, 109 (1997)

Absorption of nutrients from a raw, uncooked carrot, with its carotenoids such as lycopene, is as low as 1 to 2 percent. *"Particle size of uncooked foods is particularly important. Pureed or finely chopped vegetables yield considerably higher beta carotene absorption compared to whole or sliced raw vegetables."*

Dr. Erdman also writes that "mild heating, such as steaming, appears to improve the extractability of beta carotene from vegetables and also beta carotene availability."

The Tomato Research Council in New York City lists the best food sources of lycopene according to the amount in one ounce :[7]

Tomato ketchup	5 mg
Spaghetti sauce	5 mg
Tomato sauce	5 mg
Tomatoes, canned	3 mg
Tomato soup	3 mg
Tomato juice	3 mg
Vegetable juice	3 mg
Watermelon	1 mg
Pink grapefruit	1 mg
Vegetable beef soup	1 mg
Vegetarian vegetable soup	1 mg
Minestrone soup	1 mg

These foods and a natural lycopene supplement can promote our well-being and guard us from many degenerative diseases. *There is no disagreement that lycopene is a prostate cancer deterrent.* However, there are varying opinions as to how it reaches this objective.

Dr. Giovannucci and associates feel that more research is required to derive solid answers. However, they theorize that lycopene deters prostate cancer by means of its antioxidant function, its ability to snuff out free radicals, the militant molecules that damage cell membranes and DNA, the blueprint for cell replication.

Why this conclusion? Because byproducts of cholesterol oxidation are commonly present in prostate secretions. The Giovannucci group states that these cholesterol byproducts are cancer-causing or are indicative of oxidative stress that could influence cancer development.[8]

Another theory was presented by staff writer Janet Raloff in a *Science News* article based on interviews with various authorities.[9] These interviews point to what seems to be a paradox -- the fact that female hormones may be a major factor in causing the male ailment, prostate cancer.

Specifically, estrogen, one of the most suspect and best characterized risk factors for breast cancer, second among causes of cancer deaths in United States women, may, indeed, contribute to prostate cancer, the leading male malignancy.

Newer breast cancer research suggests that both cancers may, in part, grow from the same root: damage to DNA by estrogen. The basic evidence that seems to substantiate this provocative theory is that in prostate cancer, extensive oxidation has taken place in the precise areas where tumors form.

Raloff writes that this damage accelerates with age, along with the incidence of cancer. Shuk-mei Ho, an endocrine oncologist at Tufts University (Medford, Massachusetts), indicates that perhaps there should be a shift in research away from the male hormone testosterone in prostate cancer. Her studies suggest that hormones and their interrelationships can exert unexpected influences on human tissue.

Ho and other researchers are beginning to discover that the "hostile, free radical-laden environment that hormones might foster in the prostate could go a long way in explaining cancer's development there," writes Raloff.

The contribution of free radicals to aging in prostate tissue has triggered the development of new and increasingly precise techniques for two eminently important purposes: achieving accurate diagnosis of prostate cancer and securing evidence of DNA damage that may be the forerunner of it.

"New findings in this area suggest that dietary and other antioxidant therapies may hold great promise for curbing this scourge," writes Raloff.

The muscular prostate gland that encircles the urethra, a tube through which urine is discharged from the bladder, enlarges and tightens like a noose around the urethra, making urinating difficult -- sometimes painful -- or impossible.

Testosterone and other male sex hormones (androgens) contribute to prostate growth and cancer. However, these are not solely to blame, Raloff was told by Joachim G. Liehr, a pharmacologist at the University of Texas Medical Branch in Galveston.

Liehr highlights the critical fact that, if androgens alone were the major cause of prostate cancer, "young men of 18 or 20 at the peak of androgen production should be developing this disease."

However, this is not the case, inasmuch as prostate cancer strikes men in middle to old age when testosterone concentrations are decreasing. In contrast, men's estrogen production does not decrease, Liehr emphasized. It may even increase a bit, causing a dramatic shift in the ratio of testosterone to estrogen, a reversal he feels may foster cancer.

Researcher Maarten Bosland, of New York University Medical Center in Tuxedo, thinks along similar lines, and his thoughts are founded on some revealing animal studies.

First, Bosland administered estrogen to young castrated rats -- those unable to secrete testosterone and other male hormones -- in amounts present in their female counterparts. Not one of these rats developed prostate cancer.

Next he restored the missing testosterone to another group of young castrated rats, and between 20 and 30 percent developed prostate cancer in time. However, devastating results followed his administration of estrogen and testosterone. Almost 100 percent of the animals soon manifested prostate cancer!

Commenting on these results, Liehr theorized that the estrogen was bathing the prostate in chemicals resulting from the breakdown of estrogen, a biochemical process that triggers the release of free radicals.

In studies with animal cells in test tubes, Liehr discovered that estrogen in female reproductive tissues such as the uterus and breast is converted into a compound that is "a potent source of free radicals."

Most estrogen breakdown products degrade to harmless compounds. However, this specific one does not, so it accumulates to high and health-hazardous concentrations. Liehr also believes something similar happens to estrogen in the prostate. On the supposition that this is true, the Liehr theory could well describe the origin of cancer in prostates as men age.

Ho accepts that this process could take place. However, she insists there's more to the story --that oxidative damage takes place in cell metabolism with the constant use of oxygen and nutrients to create energy and heat.

Researcher William E. Nelson and associates, of the Johns Hopkins Medical Institute in Baltimore, found that enzymes that cause the production of protective antioxidants in cells failed to function in every sample of cancerous prostate tissue they examined.

A study of five antioxidant enzymes in the prostates of elderly rats by Ho and associates revealed a decline in their production as the rats aged. This left the animals increasingly vulnerable to free radical attacks, showing between 500 and 700 times more free radical damage in their prostates than in those of young animals.

Biochemist Donald C. Malms, of the Pacific Northwest Research Foundation in Seattle, indicated to writer, Janet Raloff that free radical damage in animals and men is made on cellular DNA.

No better evidence exists in favor of supplementing with antioxidants than in the research cited in Raloff's *Science News* story. (A great deal more about antioxidants and free radicals will follow.)

CHAPTER 2

SPECIAL PROTECTION FOR WOMEN

LYCOPENE OFFERS MANY BENEFITS

Most popular writings feature research showing benefits of lycopene to men or to both sexes, to the neglect of those benefits exclusive to women. However, there are specific lycopene benefits for women, so this sin of omission needs correction.

A research team at the University of Illinois at Chicago found that lycopene helps women guard against cervical intra-epithelial neoplasia, (CIN), tumorous tissue growth in the cervix, a necklike opening of the uterus.[1]

High levels of lycopene in the diet and in the blood protected against CIN. Women with lower lycopene intakes and blood levels were more susceptible to CIN.

In a paper entitled "Natural Antioxidants and Food Quality in Atherosclerosis and Cancer Prevention," biochemist Jorma T. Kumpulainen, of the Agricultural Research Centre in Finland, writes that factors other than beta carotene, present in diets rich with vegetables and fruit, act as cancer preventive agents.[2]

"Several epidemiological studies of patients suffering from various malignancies have suggested a cancer-preventive role for lycopene."

Relative to CIN, serum lycopene reveals a strong blocking tendency. The higher the blood levels of lycopene, the less chance of this type of cancer developing.

"No such results were obtained for the other tested carotenoids," writes Kumpulainen. "A low level of serum lycopene was also observed in patients who subsequently developed urinary and pancreatic cancers. Serum was collected from 25,802 persons in Washington County, Maryland, and kept frozen . . . for more than 12 years. The results showed that serum levels of lycopene and selenium were lower than those of matched controls."

Effectiveness of lycopene in anti-cancer roles has been demonstrated in experiments in vitro (in test-tubes) and in vivo (in living organisms), states Kumpulainen.

THE GREAT INHIBITOR

While public awareness, early detection, and new innovative treatments have held the death rate from breast cancer somewhat in check, the incidence of this disease continues to grow at an alarming rate. Over the past fifty years occurances of breast cancer have more than doubled. It is estimated that in the United States there is a new case of breast cancer being diagnosed every three minutes.

Increase in breast cancer incidence in the western world

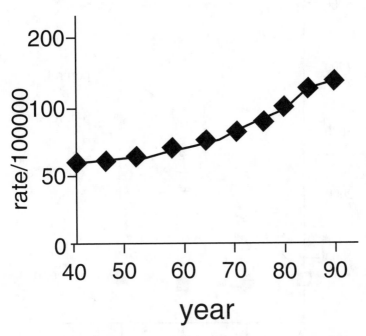

Adapted from Marshal E. Science. 259, 109 - 1993

Lycopene turned out to be a powerhouse inhibitor of the growth of breast, endometrium (inner lining of the uterus) and lung cancer cells. This is especially important because there is an increasing incidence of each of these cancers. The effectiveness of lycopene depended upon the dosage. However, *lycopene was observed to be a much stronger cancer inhibitor than either beta or alpha carotene -- 10 times stronger,* writes Kumpulainen.

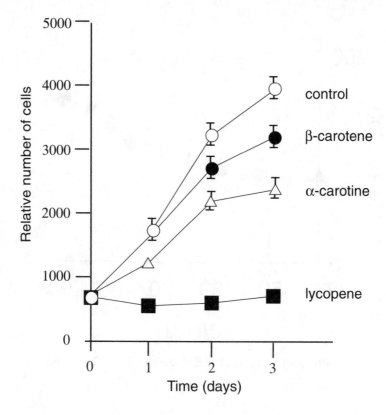

The effect of lycopene on endometrial cancer cell growth is faster than that of α-carotine and β-carotene

A ten-fold greater concentration of alpha and beta carotene than lycopene was needed to stop the growth of a certain type of breast cancer cell: MCF-7. Lycopene acted much faster than the two other carotenes in blocking the multiplication of these cancer cells --within 24 hours of incubation, compared with 48 to 72 hours for alpha and beta carotene.

Lycopene appears to inhibit cancer in two ways: by preventing its DNA synthesis and also by suppressing cell growth. Kumpulainen points out that other researchers have also demonstrated lycopene's ability to block glioma cells: cancer of the brain.

Such experiments were performed with animals, not merely in test tubes. Lycopene inhibited glioma cells transplanted in rats. Kumpulainen extended in vitro tests of various carotenoids relative to the start and spread of breast tumors in rats. He and co-workers selected the DMBA-induced rat tumor as an ideal model for studying hormone-dependent human breast cancer. Tumor growth rate is easily manipulated by estrogens and other hormones, he says.

DMBA is one of the most powerful cancer producing agents. Carotenoid treatment began two weeks before the DMBA tumors were induced. The experiment was repeated three times with 40 rats used in each phase.

Lycopene reduced the number of tumors, while beta carotene had no statistically significant effect. Tumors in the beta carotene group were larger than those treated with lycopene or even those in controls. The researchers regarded the difference in tumor size as statistically significant.

SUPPRESSED BREAST TUMORS

A later study cited by researcher Joseph Levy and associates at Ben-Gurion University of the Negev in Israel reveals that lycopene suppressed spontaneous breast tumors in a breed of mice particularly susceptible to such cancers: SHN virgin mice.[3]

Describing results of this study in *Anti-Cancer Drugs*, Japanese researchers state that one of the key roles of lycopene is normalizing tumor cells.[4]

The effect of lycopene, α-carotine and β-carotene on the growth of human mammary cancer cells

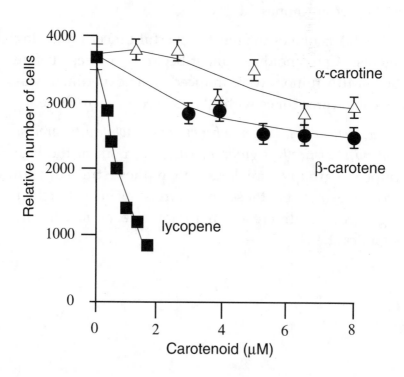

Tomato Power

Also of interest with respect to lycopene as an inhibitor of breast and endometrial cancer is its ability to block the biochemical factor IGF autocrine system, a stimulant to cancer growth. Although more investigation is needed to learn exactly how lycopene copes with breast, endometrial and lung cancers, various researchers have reasonable theories on the subject.

Acknowledging its antioxidant abilities, James Balch, M.D., in his book *The Superantioxidants*, sums up his in-depth studies of lycopene's cancer-preventive abilities [5]

"It appears that lycopene interferes with cancer cell communications so that both cell growth and cell movement were delayed in breast, lung and endometrial cancer cells . . . Lycopene increases cell differentiation, the process by which cells in the human body become specialized as liver, muscle or heart cells, among others."

There is a clear-cut advantage in using lycopene as a cancer-preventive. It induces no side effects that are so common to conventional chemotherapeutic agents.

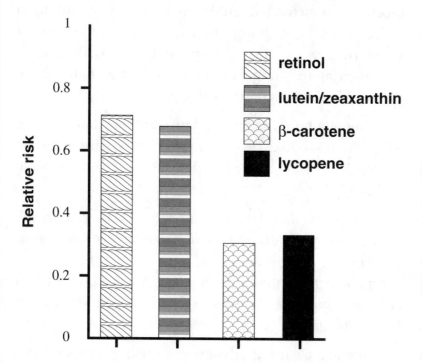

Relative risk of breast cancer is inversely associated with carotenoid adipose tissue level

Legend:
- retinol
- lutein/zeaxanthin
- β-carotene
- lycopene

Adapted from Zhang et as.Am. J.Clin. Nutr, 66, 626, - 1997

Lycopene may seem like something new among nutrients. Yet it has been well known since 1959 as a substance with possibilities for protecting individuals from exposure to radiation. A researcher named L. Ernster and co-workers injected lycopene into mice that were then exposed to lethal irradiation. The survival rate of the injected mice was increased compared with that of controls.[6]

More recently, research in this area has been revived. Much skin cancer in women and men is due to exposure to the sun's ultraviolet rays. A study by researchers at the Human Nutrition Center in Boston indicates that lycopene may protect the skin from such radiation, and consequently, from skin cancer.[7]

Caucasian women averaging 66 years of age participated in this study. At the beginning of the study, the amount of lycopene in the skin and blood were comparable to, or even greater than, the amount of beta carotene there. One day after lycopene was taken, the amount of this nutrient in the blood increased by 127 percent and remained elevated for five days.

Beta carotene in the skin increased just slightly. The intake of beta carotene did not alter the amount of lycopene in the blood or skin. However, when the skin was exposed to ultraviolet light, lycopene in the skin was significantly reduced. Beta carotene was reduced slightly or not at all.

Human Nutrition Research Center scientists observed that carotenoids are used up as they protect body tissues. Therefore, they feel *lycopene may well be an important defender against skin damage from sunlight.*

LYCOPENE HELPED ANIMALS SURVIVE

That this opinion may be correct is brought out in a Russian study of animals.[8] Given lycopene and then exposed to a lethal dose of radiation, many of these animals survived. The control animals didn't.

Some researchers theorize that lycopene guards us not only as an antioxidant, but also as a protector of immune system cells, maintaining their structure and the ability to do their work. A strong immune system fends off much disease, increasing hardiness. So, in this sense, lycopene contributes not only to promoting good health, but also to life-extension.

Chapter 3

Versatile Defender

Lycopene Guards Against Cancers, Heart Attacks and Toxic Pollutants

Hooked on cigarettes and unable to quit, more and more individuals shop at nutrition centers for supplements to protect themselves from emphysema and lung cancer.

When they order vitamins A, C and E, they are buying a measure of security. However, when they ask for beta carotene as the most likely carotenoid/antioxidant to be of help, they may be ordering the wrong product, as several studies show.

In a publication entitled "Lycopene is a More Potent Inhibitor of Human Cancer Cell Proliferation Than Either A-Carotene and B-Carotene," Dr. Joseph Levy and associates in the department of clinical biochemistry at Ben-Gurion University of the Negev state that this is so.[1]

Another study, "Dietary Factors in Lung Cancer Prognosis," by M.T. Goodman et al; presented in the European journal *Cancer* explains the following:

"Beta carotene-rich foods such as papaya, sweet potato, mango and yellow-orange vegetables showed little influence on the survival of lung cancer patients." The authors concluded that beta carotene intake before diagnosis of lung cancer does not affect the progression of the disease.

"In contrast, a tomato-rich diet which contributes only small amounts of beta carotene to the total carotenoid intake had a strong positive relationship with survival, particularly in women."[2]

ENEMY OF LUNG CANCER

Speaking to a recent American Association for Cancer Research meeting in San Diego, Jean Ford, Ph.D., of Columbia University, announced that after examining 204 people -- half with lung cancer -- *blood levels of lycopene were significantly lower in cancer patients than in healthy controls.* After accounting for smoking, Dr. Ford and associates found that those with lowest blood levels of lycopene have triple the risk of cancer than those with high levels.[4]

"This is a preliminary report, but it raises questions about whether there are dietary risk factors that we need to take a closer look at for lung cancer," she stated.

In a letter to the editor of *Nature Medicine*, biochemist F. Bohm, of Charite Hospital, Humboldt Universitate, Berlin, and associates, indicate that lycopene is a better protector against the harm from cigarette smoke and other air pollutants than beta carotene.[5]

Numerous reports reveal that harmful air pollutants are not always as visible as smog that blankets major industrial cities. Therefore, it is a mistake to assume that what appears to be clean air actually is clean, and to take no protective action. Nitrogen dioxide is a major air pollutant, and cigarette smoke contains high concentrations of nitric oxide. Reacting with oxygen, these substances produce hydrogen radicals, peroxy radicals and nitrous acid.

Bohm and coauthors write, "Nitric oxide radicals can extract hydrogen from linoleic and linolenic acids and trigger peroxidation both in vitro and in vivo, causing cell membrane damage. Free radicals survive long enough in fresh tobacco smoke to enter lungs."

Further, based on their experiments, the authors find that lycopene better protects lymphocyte cells from nitrogen free radicals than beta carotene. Therefore, they write, *"Our results suggest an anti-cancer strategy in which lycopene should be considered as an alternative to beta carotene in intervention trials."*

In a fascinating study of comparative protective values of beta carotene and lycopene, Bohm and associates irradiated human lymphocyte cells and a nitric oxide-generating solution to 300 laser pulses.

These cells, unprotected by carotenoid, showed a death rate of 25.3 percent in one experiment and 23.6 per cent in another. When cells were coated with beta carotene, dead cells were reduced to 7.4 percent. When they were coated with lycopene, there were only 2.8 percent dead cells.

On increasing the radiation strength, the cell kill with no carotenoids present was 51.6 percent and 74.3 percent respectively. This was reduced to 14.6 for beta carotene-coated cells and 9.1 for lycopene coated cells.

"Our results show that both carotenoids are effective protectors of lymphocyte cells from nitric oxide radical damage, but that lycopene is at least twice as effective as beta carotene," conclude the writers. "The major practical result is that lycopene is shown to be a more efficient protector against a major toxic component of polluted air and cigarette smoke . . . than beta carotene. Thus, anti-cancer trials should be extended to lycopene, especially when smokers are involved."

Another researcher reports an interesting reaction of lycopene to a high intake of alcohol.[6] Dr. Elizabeth Johnson reveals that heavy drinkers deplete blood levels of lycopene. Non-drinkers and moderate drinkers have far higher levels of lycopene than alcoholics. However, after three weeks off alcohol, heavy drinkers slowly begin to build back their lycopene blood levels.

Protective effects of lycopene go beyond smoking and drinking. Dr. S. Franceschi, of the University of Milan, revealed that *people who ate seven or more servings per week of tomato-based products had 60 percent less chance of developing colon, mouth, rectal and stomach cancers than those who didn't.*[7]

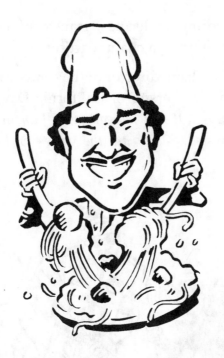

Model depiction of oxidation.

How does lycopene guard us against threats to our health? Numerous researchers suggest that it strengthens the immune system and protects us from the negative aspects of oxygen. Oxygen is both a giver and a taker. It supports life and undermines it.

Oxygen in every one of our cells is needed for metabolizing ("burning") our food ("fuel") to develop energy and warmth. Metabolizing goes on every instant of the day and night.

Oxidation causes molecules to lose an electron. This changes them into free radicals, militant molecules that multiply geometrically and forcibly seize an electron from neighboring molecules, transforming them into free radicals, starting a chain reaction.

Dr. Mary N. Haan, director of the center for Aging and Health at the University of California-Davis School of Medicine, says, *"If free radicals were human beings, they would be arrested. They are the gangs or looters in our bodies."*[8]

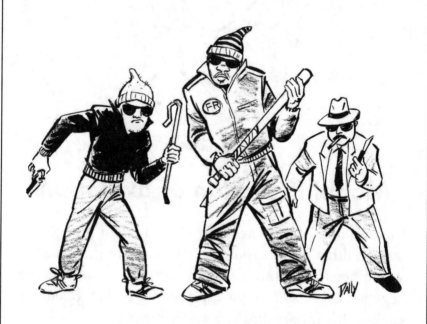

A philosopher created the expression, "The best things in life are free." Obviously, he knew nothing about free radicals. Free radicals would be numerous and undermining enough even if they resulted only from our metabolic processes.

THEY COME AT US FROM EVERYWHERE

Unfortunately, there are many more sources. Free radicals bombard us in solar radiation, X-rays, electrical appliances, smog -- an estimated 10,000 pollutants, including cigarette smoke, impure drinking water and some 3,000 food additives. All forms of stress create free radicals -- mental, emotional and physical -- everything from ordinary physical exercise to gruelling marathons, and muscle-cramping manual labor. So do burns, sickness, accidents and even the process of body hormones maintaining their proper ratios and balances.

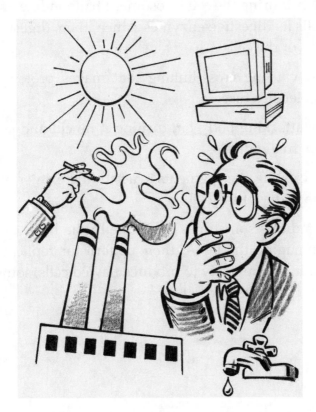

During a recent meeting of the American Academy of Anti-Aging Medicine in Las Vegas, Denham Harman, M.D., who, in the mid-1950s discovered the free radical theory, stated that he is "more convinced than ever that free radicals are the cause of most, if not all degenerative diseases and accelerate the aging process." [9]

Free radicals cause damage in five ways, he says:

1. By attacking cell membranes, damaging their integrity and flexibility, making it difficult for them to absorb nutrients and oxygen and discharge wastes.

2. By rupturing the cell lysosome, a balloon-like object that spills its digestive enzymes which, then, digest critical parts of the cell.

3. By causing cross-linking that makes proteins or DNA molecules fuse.

4. By attacking body fat, turning it rancid and creating more free radicals.

5. By causing age-pigments to accumulate, interfering with chemistry of the cell.

Free radicals sometimes penetrate to the heart of the cells, damaging the DNA, their pattern for replication, and making them likely to produce flawed cells, some of which may evolve into cancer.

ANTIOXIDANTS FOR THE DEFENSE

The body makes antioxidants that quench free radicals, otherwise there would be a runaway free radical rampage that would destroy the body. We take in more antioxidants in food. Still there may be too many free radicals for existing antioxidants to handle, so many of us take antioxidant supplements.

In a review paper, "Oxidants, Antioxidants and the Degenerative Diseases of Aging," Bruce Ames, Ph.D., division of biochemistry and molecular biology, University of California, Berkeley, explains our defense system against free radicals.[10]

When cell DNA is oxygen-damaged, certain enzymes perform chemical surgery, excising injured parts and repairing the damage.

"We estimate that the number of oxidative hits to DNA per cell per day is about 100,000 in the rat and about 10,000 in the human. DNA repair enzymes efficiently remove most, but not all, of the lesions formed," writes Dr. Ames.

"Oxidative lesions in DNA accumulate with age, so that by the time the rat is old (2 years), it has had about 2 million DNA lesions per cell, which is about twice that in a young rat. Mutations accumulate with age . . . "

Dr. Ames states that *smoking is a major oxidative stress as well as a source of mutagens and "contributes to about one-third of U.S. cancer, about one-quarter U.S. heart disease and about 400,000 premature deaths per year in the U.S."*

Considered one of the most powerful antioxidants, lycopene also offers a stout defense against cell damage from the toxic chemical carbon tetrachloride, often used for spot cleaning in dry cleaning establishments and in homes.[11]

When lycopene (along with other carotenoids) was added to rat liver cells that had been exposed to carbon tetrachloride, it reduced cell injury.

MORE EFFECTIVE AGAINST CANCER

Speaking at an an Antioxidant Conference in the United Kingdom, biochemist Simon Martin told conferees that research already shows that *lycopene is more effective than other carotenoids in the prevention of cancer and may have a role in cancer treatment.*[12]

"Results will revolutionize current thinking on carotene antioxidants, based on research almost exclusively carried out with beta-carotene. It will come as a surprise to many that beta-carotene, valuable though it is, is only a small part of the story."

Simon Martin then saluted Dr. Fred Khachik, a USDA researcher on carotenoids since 1983, for his breakthrough studies that revealed for the first time that lycopene and lutein protect mainly by being powerful antioxidants.

It was Dr. Khachik's team that discovered "that part of the reason lycopene is so effective is that it is broken down into metabolites which are even more protective than lycopene itself."

Researcher Martin told the congress that lycopene's defense system goes beyond its antioxidant function. Lycopene also improves detoxification and is known to "switch on the mechanism that normally tells cells to stop growing a mechanism that goes wrong in cancer cells."

And lycopene's versatile defense system also extends beyond protecting against various cancers, to biochemical insurance against heart and artery disease.

Tomato Power

Chapter 4

Insurance for Heart, Eyes and Brain

Antioxidants Protect Life, Vision and Ability to Think

It may come as a shock to many individuals, but biochemist Richard A. Passwater, Ph.D., feels that even cholesterol-sensitive people should realize that "antioxidant protection is more important than cholesterol level.[1]

"Don't concentrate on the minor problem and ignore the major factor," he advises in his segment of a book written by many authorities, *The Nutrition Superbook: The Antioxidants*, edited by Jean Barilla and published by Keats Publishing, Inc.

Stressing the importance of taking vitamin E regularly to guard against heart disease, Dr. Passwater explains that heart attack is a two-step process.

Foam cells, macrophages, stick to the artery lining. These are Pac Man-like immune system cells that gobble up bacteria, toxins and other foreign matter as well as oxidized low density lipoprotein (LDL), considered the bad cholesterol. This initial plaque attracts other plaque on the intima, the smooth artery interior. As this buildup grows, the artery narrows, and blood flow to the heart muscle decreases. Blood platelets are often damaged as they squeeze through. This makes the blood sticky and more prone to clot at the plaqued area.

Antioxidants can prevent the first step: the forming of plaque. They protect the artery interior from becoming injured, prevent blood platelets from clumping, and lessen their stickiness so they are less likely to adhere to the intima.

Michael Aviram, Ph.D., and Bianca Fuhrman, in a publication "Lycopene and Atherosclerosis," explain that the macrophage cholesterol accumulation and foam cell formation are the initial signs of atherosclerosis (artery blockage).[2]

Low density lipoprotein in and of itself is not dangerous. It becomes so when oxidized. Dietary antioxidants can block this process. Dr. Aviram used various nutrients (including antioxidants) to stop this process: vitamins E and C, the trace mineral selenium, olive oil, licorice root extract, beta carotene and lycopene.

"Both lycopene and beta carotene inhibited the oxidation of linoleic acid (the major fatty acid in LDL) by up to 51 percent and 29 percent, respectively," he writes.

HOW ATHEROSCLEROSIS STARTS

Arterial wall macrophages that are loaded with oxidized LDL-derived cholesterol during early atherosclerosis, can oxidize LDL. The researchers studied the effect of mediated oxidation of LDL. Some macrophages or LDL were enriched with lycopene, others with beta carotene.

Role of Oxidized Lipoproteins in Atherogenesis

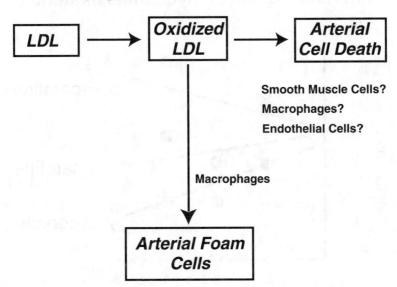

Endothelial Cells
Smooth Muscle Cells
Macrophages

LDL → Oxidized LDL → Arterial Cell Death

Smooth Muscle Cells?
Macrophages?
Endothelial Cells?

Macrophages

Arterial Foam Cells

Enrichment with lycopene led to reduction of LDL oxidation by 68 percent. Enrichment with beta carotene led to just a 46 percent reduction of oxidation.

In human blood plasma, lycopene and beta carotene are the major carotenoids, with lycopene number one in that it is 50 percent of circulating carotenoids. *Lycopene was shown to be far superior to any other carotenoid in quenching singlet oxygen, one of the most vicious of free radicals.*

Any reasonable preventive measures for reducing the chance of heart attack are worthy of consideration, because there is the possibility of danger beyond the usual physical and emotional devastation.

Lycopene adipose tissue level is associated with reduced risk of myocaridal infarction

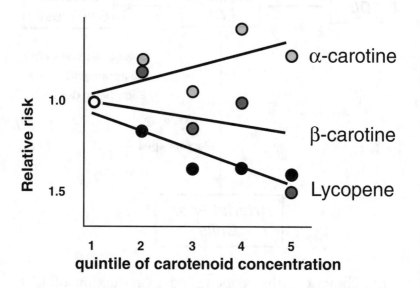

Adapted from Kohlmeier et al Am J Epidemiol, 146, 618, - 1997

A recent issue of the University of Texas, Houston, Health Science Center *Lifetime Health Letter* contains the warning by Howard Fillet, M.D., a professor of geriatrics, medicine and neurobiology at Mount Sinai School of Medicine in New York, that a heart attack may damage the brain.[3]

Some heart attack patients attribute loss of ability to think effectively and remember to aging or to

Alzheimer's disease. The real culprit could be a condition called vascular dementia. As its name indicates, vascular dementia (decline in intellectual function) is caused by blood vessel disorders resulting from a heart attack, high blood pressure or a stroke.

As people age, vascular dementia becomes more common, says Dr. Fillet, indicating that in the very old -- age 85 or older -- vascular dementia is at least as common as Alzheimer's disease and is often misdiagnosed as that.

Not a new ailment, vascular dementia is now viewed in a different light. Until recently, it was considered in a narrow context: the consequence of a stroke or as the accumulated damage of many transient strokes, mini-strokes associated only with temporary impairment.

Today, doctors take the broader view that dementia may be caused not only by a stroke, but by other arterial problems that affect the flow of blood to the brain. Most forms of vascular dementia are treatable, protecting the brain from further loss of function.

BRAINS IN MOTHBALLS?

When their thinking processes slow down and memory deserts them, some individuals jump to the conclusion that they have some form of dementia or even Alzheimer's disease. This is sad, because these conditions are often brought on by the individual himself or herself due to mental stagnation.

Noted neuroanatomist Marian Diamond, Ph.D., of the University of California at Berkeley, says that brains are only large clumps of nerve cells. *Nerve cells were created to be stimulated. Use them or lose them.*[4]

Research performed by Maria G. Boorsalis and David Snowdon, Ph.D., professor of preventive medicine at the Sanders-Brown Center on Aging at the University of Kentucky, bears out Dr. Diamond's findings.[5]

A continuing study of 88 aged nuns of the School Sisters of Notre Dame in Mankato, Minnesota, shows that those who stay mentally and physically active live longer, remain healthier and think and remember better. [6]

These individuals are in their eighties and nineties, with several over 100. And this is where lycopene comes in. Sisters with or without dementia or Alzheimer's disease who have the highest blood levels of lycopene retain their memory, a positive disposition, and the ability to care for themselves and their hygienic needs longer than those with low levels.

The Borsalis team also reveals important information about acute phase response and its relation to carotenoid concentration. Acute phase response is medical jargon for reaction to stress. What happens to blood plasma levels of lycopene and other antioxidants when a person is stressed?

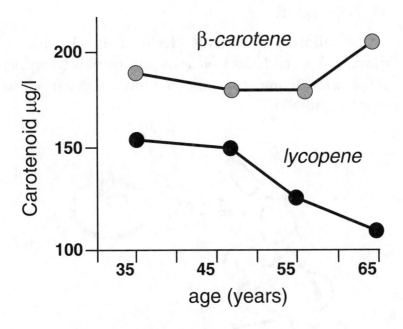

Age-dependent changes in antioxidant plasma levels

Carotenoid µg/l

β-carotene

lycopene

200

150

100

35   45   55   65

age (years)

Adapted from: Buiatti, et al. Int. J. Cancer 65, 317 (1996)

ANTIOXIDANTS TO THE RESCUE

Many studies show that antioxidants decrease as they protect tissue damage from oxidation. Oxidative damage can change gene expression, produce mutagens, cause cell membrane damage and reduce levels of anti-oxidants circulating in the blood.

Types of stress that brought on acute phase response in the nunnery were not necessarily extreme: uncomplicated orthopedic surgery, gingivitis (inflamed gums), insulin dependent diabetes, Paget's disease, and, among others, bronchitis.

The following nutrients declined in the blood: vitamins A, C, and E as well as the carotenoids lycopene, alpha carotene and beta carotene indicating a need to supplement them.

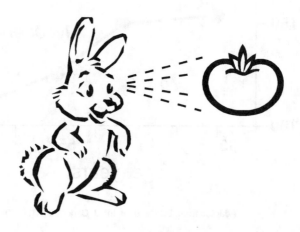

Tomatoes are good for the eyes, too.

Other kinds of stress bring on an ailment, not uncommon to the nuns, that occurs mainly in elderly individuals: Age-Related Macular Degeneration (ARMD), a condition that may cause blindness.

Exposure to the harmful frequencies of sunlight, as well as to oxygen over the years, endangers the macula, a small, yellowish area, the true center of sight at the back of the retina. High blood and tissue levels of vitamin E and lycopene seem to delay or even to fend off macular degeneration. This was demonstrated in a recent mass study.[7]

A MISUNDERSTANDING

Called the Beaver Dam (Wisconsin) Eye Study, this research project involved 170 volunteers with more severe stages of early and late ARMD. Some scientific investigation indicates that lutein and zeaxanthin -- due to their yellowish color -- are the major players in preventing age-related macular degeneration.

However, the lead scientist in the study, Julie A. Meres-Perlman, Ph.D., says, "No. Levels of the carotenoids that compose macular pigment -- lutein with zeaxanthin -- in the serum were unrelated to ARMD."

What was discovered is that, in the wet form of macular degeneration, called the "exudative" type, "average levels of vitamin E were lower."

Dr. Meres-Perlman found lycopene, the most abundant carotenoid in the blood serum, to be the key antioxidant that guards against ARMD. *Persons with levels of lycopene in the lowest quintile "were twice as likely to have age-related macular degeneration," she states.*

Here is the conclusion of the study:

"Very low levels of one (lycopene) but no other dietary carotenoids or tocopherols were related to ARMD. Lower levels of vitamin E in subjects with exudative macular degeneration compared with controls may be explained by lower levels of serum lipids."

Even though lycopene is not highly concentrated in the macula, it is a potent force in the eye, writes Meres-Perlman. This may be due to "its greater ability to quench singlet oxygen, a reactive species in the eye."

Another point made by the study is this:

Because the retina is highly susceptible to damage by exposure to light and oxygen, the antioxidants vitamin C and vitamin E -- as well as carotenoids -- have been protective of the retina in experimental animals.

Further, lycopene was shown to be at least twice as effective an antioxidant as beta carotene in protecting blood lymphocytes from free radical damage. *The versatility it [lycopene] shows in protecting us in various areas of the body is truly remarkable.*[8]

CHAPTER 5
IMPORTANCE OF TESTING

Authorities Cite the Need to Know Antioxidant Levels

On the surface, it seems like a mystery! Obviously, free radicals age us and threaten us with a medical book full of degenerative diseases, making it a must to have an army of antioxidants powerful enough to keep them under control.

Yet how do we know if there are enough antioxidant soldiers in us? We can only guess. And that's a risky way to operate our personal Department of Defense.

For many years, eminent antioxidant authorities have urged laboratories to offer a panel of blood tests to determine the status of antioxidants. Among them are Denham Harman, M.D., father of the free radical theory,[1] and William A. Pryor, Ph.D., one of the foremost authorities on antioxidants and head of biomedical research at Louisiana State University at Baton Rouge.

In a personal communication, Dr. Pryor said that blood level testing should be conducted just as we measure for blood cholesterol.[2] The testing should actually do two things: (1) determine the amount of damage caused by free radicals --what he calls "oxidative stress status" (OSS) -- and (2) reveal the kind and amounts of antioxidants in our blood serum.[1]

"Extensive oxidative damage and low levels of neutralizing antioxidants would put the patient in a high risk category, and he or she would then know how much to increase his or her intake of antioxidants," said Dr. Pryor.

Remember, in the opening paragraph of the previous chapter, Dr. Richard Passwater told us that "antioxidant protection is more important than cholesterol level," and that we shouldn't concentrate on the minor problem and ignore the major factor.

Unfortunately, conventional doctors are still hung up on the cholesterol theory and may take additional conditioning to come around to the Harman/Pryor/Passwater vantage point.

PLEASE MAKE THEM LEGIBLE, DOCTOR!

Doctors must write prescriptions in order for patients to have an antioxidant test. Preventive or holistic medical doctors are the most likely to write them, while conventional doctors are less likely to do this. Therefore, it is time for patients to become impatient and take the initiative.

Dr. Richard Passwater says "We can't all live to 100. However, with whole foods and proper nutritional supplementation -- including antioxidants -- we can live far longer and protect ourselves from the pain, limitation and inconvenience of unnecessary illness and upgrade the quality of our lives." [3]

The book *Life Extenders and Memory Boosters* by multiple authorities (Health Quest Publications) shows the critical importance of proper antioxidant supplementation by noting that the National Institutes of Health is completing a $17 million, five-year study to learn specifics about how antioxidants help prevent cancer and heart disease.[4]

Without indicating the particular free radical fighters involved, this book highlights striking accomplishments of antioxidants. *A University of Wisconsin study demonstrated that antioxidants can prolong human life by at least 14 percent.*

ENCOURAGING EVIDENCE

A double-blind animal experiment by Denham Harman, M.D., at the University of Nebraska, showed that animals given antioxidants had virtually no tumors when they died. Control subjects had many.

A World Health Organization study revealed that men in 16 European cities with the lowest levels of antioxidants in their blood were far more likely candidates to suffer from fatal heart attacks than those with the highest.

The link was so strong that researchers ruled out "cholesterol levels as a contributing reason for this startling difference between the highest and lowest antioxidants in their bodies."

One study demonstrated that memory loss could be overcome with antioxidants by reversing free radical-related cellular damage.

Further, this book states that antioxidants may be able to hold back diseases "like Parkinson's, stroke, heart disease, cataract and some cancers."

Aware of these facts and, supported by appeals from eminent authorities for cooperation, one laboratory began blood test panels for antioxidants even before there was a demand from patients: Pantox Laboratories in San Diego 1-800 726-8698.[5]

The founder and director of research and development at Pantox is Charles A. Thomas, Jr., Ph.D., a molecular biologist who earned his Ph.D in physical chemistry at Harvard University and has researched the structure of viral nucleic acid for about 20 years.

Dr. Thomas had been a professor of biophysics at Johns Hopkins and a professor of biological chemistry at Harvard Medical School before joining the cell biology department at the Scripps Research Foundation and then forming his own laboratory.

If Dr. Thomas' present work seems to be unrelated to his former activities, he says there's definitely a connection.

"My focus on the replication and transcription of nucleic acids directed me to think about how DNA was damaged and how mutations come about. What are the damaging agents and what are their sources?

"The most mutagenic agents are oxygen free radicals generated by normal biochemistry, plus dozens of environmental sources such as solar and man-made radiation, smog, polluted water, pesticides and food additives."

IMPRESSIVE ASSOCIATES

Added to its distinguished founder-director, Pantox has an impressive list of founding scientists and consultants: Helmut Sies, M.D., Peter Cerutti, M.D., Ph.D, Lester Packer, Ph.D., Fred Gey, Ph.D., Christian Mende, M.D., Jeffrey Fisher, M.D., Mark McCarty, Bruce N. Ames, Ph.D., Balz Frey, Ph.D., Eugene Weinberg, Ph.D., Mark Macozzi, M.D., Ph.D., and Kilmer McCully, M.D.

As for Pantox's panel of antioxidants for assay, there are 20 in two categories: (1) lipid soluble substances -- lycopene, beta and alpha carotene, among them -- and (2) water soluble nutrients.

"New antioxidants are constantly being discovered and as substantial research validates their importance, we'll add them to our panel," says Dr. Thomas.

"Nature has given us an antioxidant defense system. Its abilities vary from individual to individual. It is our responsibility to maintain and improve this system," Dr. Thomas states.

"However, disease and malnutrition -- even among supposedly well-nourished people -- mental and physical trauma and just normal aging impair our antioxidant defenses. What I'm saying is especially true of older people who often have very poor diets and do not absorb the antioxidant micronutrients they should for optimum protection."

MUCH MORE SCIENTIFIC

Asked what recommendations Pantox makes if a patient is low on just about every item on the panel, Dr. Thomas answered, "We recommend significantly higher levels of antioxidants in the form of supplements. *Supplementation almost always elevates blood serum levels of critically needed antoxidants.* It represents a vast leap ahead of just supplementing antioxidants according to guess and hunch."

How often should a patient have an antioxidant blood profile?

"Assuming that the person is deficient in most or all the needed antioxidants, we suggest a program of supplementation. When this is followed, we suggest a repeat test four to six months later. Once the patient shows a good profile, we recommend an annual biochemical checkup," he said.

How does Pantox work?

"We are a CLIA-approved reference laboratory licensed in the state of California," replied Dr. Thomas. "At this point, we have measured Pantox profiles in more than 3,000 blood samples.

"This is accepted procedure. The Pantox profile must be ordered by a licensed practitioner in the state where the blood sample is drawn. Most of our orders come from physicians, but some come from other practitioners, as well."

What is the cost?

"At this time, it is $250, if payment is sent with the specimen. Clinically, our antioxidant profiles are used in two ways: (1) as preventive diagnostic screens and (2) as part of diagnostic and treatment protocols.

"When a valid ICD-9 diagnostic code is included on the Patient Information/Requisition form, cost of the panel is considered eligible for coverage by almost all insurance plans," he stated. "We also accept Medicare assignment. Further, we bill patients (and submit insurance claims on their behalf, if their insurance information is included with the blood sample) or we bill the doctor directly, if preferred."

HELP FOR UNINITIATED DOCTORS

Inasmuch as the antioxidant panel is new to many doctors as well as patients, Pantox offers a special and helpful service.

"Any readers who would like their profiles done can phone Pantox Laboratories at 1-800 728-8696 for information. We can fill them in and send their physician or other qualified health practitioner a specimen kit, complete with simple instructions on how to package and send the blood sample," says Dr. Thomas.

"We also can recommend a doctor in their area who is familiar with our profile and how to interpret and use the results properly to upgrade patients' antioxidant levels."

Without a frame of reference, the panel would have little meaning. So Pantox compares each patient's measured values with the laboratory's large data base of values obtained from thousands of individuals.

A graph is produced to show clearly how each patient's values compare or contrast with others. A great deal of existing literature now demonstrates that patients in the upper percentiles enjoy a significantly lower rate of degenerative disease than those in lower percentiles.

"So far as I know, ours is the only profile that gives the entire antioxidant picture simultaneously -- not merely an isolated vitamin C or vitamin E assessment," says Dr. Thomas.

Although modern medicine has made substantial progress in diagnosing disease, it has taken only a few tentative steps to evaluate health and prevent disease.

"Now, for the first time we can apply state-of-the-art analytical methods to analyze health, where health is defined as reducing the risk of accumulating and progressive cellular damage that underlies the development of degenerative disease," states Dr. Thomas.

ACCENT ON PREVENTIVE MEDICINE

"Treatment of illness -- the present emphasis in medicine -- will soon be de-emphasized," he says. "The future of medicine will be mainly preventive. It will soon be as commonplace for us all to have a 'biochemical checkup' every six to 12 months as it is to have a dental checkup.

"This makes uncommonly good common sense, because it allows us to know about potential hazards before they become major problems," he states. "When the forerunners of negative conditions are discovered early, small and easy corrections can be made that permit us to avoid serious diseases.

"How much easier it is now to take the appropriate antioxidant supplements in the proper amounts to compensate for our known deficiencies and avoid often painful, limiting and life-shortening degenerative diseases."

Elaborating on the antioxidant level testing of Pantox is not intended to imply that this is the only lab conducting this test. Your doctor may know of another high quality laboratory that tests for antioxidant levels. Ask for a referral. It is not advisable to take for granted that your levels of lycopene and other antioxidants are high enough.

There is one person who can take the guesswork out of your antioxidant status. YOU!

CHAPTER 6
BEHIND THE LYCOPENE STORY

From Obscurity to Star Status

The story of lycopene may read more like fiction than fact. Yet every word is true. This carotenoid started its biochemical life in obscurity, thanks to the dazzling prominence of beta carotene, its cousin.

Every seminar on carotenoids was about beta carotene. It was almost as if no other carotenoid existed. Beta carotene had become what Robert C. Atkins, M.D., calls "the darling of the nutrition community."

Although occasional research revealed the merits of lycopene and its antioxidant powers relative to the prevention of cancer and heart disease, one recent study skyrocketed it to international attention. That study, mentioned in chapter one, was by Edward Giovannucci, M.D., and associates in the School of Public Health at Harvard .

Aside from showing that individuals who ate tomato sauce-smothered spaghetti, ketchup on hamburgers, and tomato paste-topped pizza were far less prone to develop prostate cancer, Dr. Giovannucci blasted a commonly held opinion that raw produce is usually more nutritious than cooked. He explained that the lycopene in tomatoes cooked with a little fat is best absorbed.

Suddenly lycopene became a biochemical Cinderella at the Prince's ball. Now carotenoid conferences are mainly about lycopene. And beta carotene hardly gets a dance, although it deserves better than that.

Lycopene seems to be a newly discovered supplement. However, it was actually isolated more than 125 years ago, separated, purified and described by several researchers. Its importance was dramatically demonstrated in a 1959 animal experiment by a biochemist named L. Ernster and associates.

The survival rate of irradiated mice was significantly increased when they were injected with lycopene. A related experiment revealed that an injection of lycopene also made lab animals more resistant to bacterial infection.

CAUSE OF FRUSTRATION

Researchers became excited about lycopene's apparent possibilities but were frustrated by the lack of a ready supply of lycopene for their studies.

Three visionary researchers at the Mahkteshim-Agan Ltd.'s Natural Products Division, Beer Sheva, Israel, anticipated the growing importance of, and need for, lycopene. Realizing the business opportunities in lycopene, this company established an independent daughter firm, LycoRed Natural Products Industries Ltd., of Beer Shiva, Israel. Its role was to develop a reliable and high quality source of lycopene.[1]

Tomatoes were known to have a higher lycopene content than any other vegetable or fruit and, therefore, offered the greatest promise. However, the lycopene in conventional tomatoes is relatively low.

One thing was obvious. A new breed of tomatoes would have to be created and developed to be rich in lycopene while preserving other properties in tomatoes important to LycoRed. This required in-depth study, a heavy investment of money, trial and error and seven long years.

The LycoRed Natural Products Industries scientists worked in the tradition of the late Luther Burbank, ingenious American plant experimenter who created new kinds of tomatoes, asparagus, peaches and even a spineless cactus for cattle feeding. They used novel agro-breeding techniques -- *no genetic engineering* -- to develop luscious, vine-ripened, super-red tomatoes that contained three times more lycopene than ordinary tomatoes.

ADAM WOULD HAVE BEEN TEMPTED

Selecting ideal locations with rich and fertile soil, they grew their Garden of Eden tomatoes and converted them into an industrial product.

Knowledgeable consumers justifiably fear genetically engineered vegetables and fruit that have not been researched enough to assure safety for human use. Many tend to regard eating genetically engineered produce as a form of nutritional Russian Roulette.

Informed consumers also appreciate the bonus benefits in natural supplements such as LYC-O-MATO tomato over the small amount of lycopene produced from fungi, which is not an approved and safe source.

One more towering plus of the LYC-O-MATO natural tomato lycopene comes from LycoRed Natural Product Industries' discovery and use of a guaranteed nutrient-protecting way of extracting rich lycopene without commonly used chemicals. Chemicals always leave a residue. Harmful or harmless, such chemical residues do not belong in nutritional products.

Infinite care is taken to protect this company's lycopene from high temperatures and exposure to oxygen to preserve maximum food and antioxidant values and to assure a standardized concentration of at least 6 percent. Every precaution is taken throughout the processing to protect lycopene against deterioration and to present it to the consumer in its native state.

Leading makers of nutritional supplements worldwide use the LycoRed Products Industries' tomato oleoresin as the basis for their natural lycopene. Nutrition center owners and store personnel know, or can find out, which companies' lycopene supplements contain this high quality base. For a listing of products containing lycopene see page 91.

One prominent maker of nutritional supplements has combined lycopene, lutein and zeaxanthin into a supplement meant to guard the eyes and eyesight.

Another has blended lycopene with alpha and beta carotene, cryptoxanthin, lutein and zeaxanthin, a carotenoid mixture that simulates the combination in fruits and vegetables that is calculated to deliver a one-two punch to militant free radicals.

Another prominent firm is planning to create a harmony of ginkgo biloba, garlic extract and lycopene, along with other carotenoids. The ginkgo biloba is intended to open micro circulation for more efficient delivery of blood laden with oxygen and nutrients to the body's trillions of cells.

It takes one ton of tomatoes to produce about 100 grams of pure lycopene or approximately 2 kg of oleoresin containing 6 percent lycopene. (A gram is 1/28th of an ounce.)

Lycopene extract is a natural tomato oleoresin that also contains vitamin E, beta carotene and other important phytochemicals.

OTHER USES

To assure the complete safety of the lycopene supplement, LycoRed Natural Products Industries conducted a million dollars worth of tests, according to Simon Martin in *BioMED*, an English research publication.[2] Quality costs money, time and infinite patience.

Beyond its major use as a natural tomato oleoresin and antioxidant nutritional supplement, LYC-O-MATO is also being utilized as a natural additive to commercial food products. Such products as tomato powder, concentrates, sauces and soups vary in lycopene content over a wide range, as food technologists know. However, manufacturers of these products can now standardize them by adding lycopene-rich tomato ingredients. This will broaden their market by appealing to health-conscious customers.

LycoRed Natural Products Industries Ltd. collaborates with interested food manufacturers and compounders by supplying them with technical data, scientific information and consulting.

The company offers help to food manufacturers for many possible applications of its tomato oleoresin: for soft and hard shell capsules or as an ingredient for beverages, dry mixes, sauces and miscellaneous food formulations. It also offers standardization of amounts of lycopene in tomato-based products such as ketchup, sauces, soups and concentrates. LYC-O-MATO is ideal for enriching ready-to-use tomato juice. Other applications are limited only by the imagination.

Alert and creative, LycoRed Natural Products Industries saw still another need for LYC-O-MATO -- natural coloring substance for foods, pharmaceuticals and cosmetics.

Many health-minded individuals object to foods and other products taken into their bodies or applied to them that contain artificial colors. The FDA banned all synthetic colors found to cause cancer in animal studies. Therefore, food processors have only a very limited number of colors they can apply to their products.

In addition, the approved colors are limited only to certain uses. The few remaining artificial colors on the list are under investigation as damaging to health (allergenic, mutagenic or carcinogenic) and the food containing them. So there's a strong trend toward natural coloring such as that in LYC-O-MATO.

LYC-O-MATO OVERCOMES DRAWBACKS

Until the coming of LYC-O-MATO, natural pigments were plagued by serious drawbacks, writes biochemist Zohar Nir, Ph.D., in a paper, "Lycopene From Tomatoes," where, with colleagues, he developed the brilliant red product.[3]

Most coloring substances were unstable to heat and to acidic or alkaline pH values. Some imparted offensive flavors to products and offered unstable and undependable coloring. Other natural pigments provided a severely limited color range and were effective only in high concentrations.

Lycopene coloring brought many advantages without a serious drawback that comes with beta carotene. Beta carotene is one of the few good natural colors available, but it is limited to the yellow-orange color range. However, to call beta carotene coloring "natural," is to place a severe strain on this word.

UNNATURAL "NATURAL" BETA CAROTENE

As Dr. Nir writes, "Only a small percentage of beta carotene used in various industries is, in fact, truly natural. Most of it is a 'nature identical,' chemically synthesized, all transisomer of the pigment.

"Tomato lycopene, being very similar in chemical composition to B-carotene, has all the natural advantages necessary to make it an excellent food color," he continues. "It is also stable to heat and extreme pH values encountered in food processing.

"In addition, lycopene has a much wider color range than B carotene -- from yellow through orange to red -- and is effective in very low concentrations. For example, solubilized lycopene, in the yellow/orange color range, is six to eight times more effective than beta carotene."

However, the main thrust of LYC-O-MATO remains as a nutritional supplement. It is the most plentiful carotenoid in the human blood and cannot be synthesized by the body. Therefore, it must be ingested in food and/or supplement form.

In this Age of Stress when events move at a frantic pace -- when one must do too much in too little time -- it isn't always possible to include tomato products and other lycopene-containing food in the everyday diet. Yet the need to protect body and mind from free radical assaults that contribute to degenerative diseases and a shorter lifespan goes on 24-hours a day.

It is frightening to recall the statistic offered by Dr. Bruce Ames that DNA in our trillions of cells is bombarded by as many as 10,000 hits daily.

When, for whatever reasons, diet doesn't include enough lycopene, it is comforting to know that major nutrition companies such as Twinlab, GNC, Nature's Herbs, Bronson, and others are now marketing health-insuring lycopene products based on the world's richest red tomatoes.

Tomato Power

APPENDIX A

SUPPLEMENTS CONTAINING LYCOPENE

The following is a partial list of companies that supply nutritional supplements containing lycopene. The list is not complete because new nutritional supplements incorporating lycopene are rapidly being developed in response to an increasing awareness of the health benefits of this super anti-oxidant.

TWINLAB
150 Motor Parkway
Hauppauge, NY 11788

TWINLAB®
NATURAL TOMATO LYCOPENE

One (1) Softgel capsule provides:
LYC-O-MATO™ Natural Tomato Lycopene . . . . . 10 mg

<u>TWINLAB®</u>
<u>MEN'S SOY PROSTATE PROTECTOR</u>
<u>WITH LOCOPENE</u>

Two (2) Softgel capsules provide:
LYC-O-MATO™ Natural Tomato Lycopene . . . . . 10 mg
Novasoy™ Purified Soy Extact . . . . 200 mg
   (providing 40% isoflavones)
   (providing 80 mg of isoflavones,)
   (including 39 mg of genistein,
   34 mg of diadzein, and
   7 mg of glyciten)
Natural Vitamin E. . . . . 400 IU
Natural Vitamin D (from Cod Liver Oil) . . . . 400 IU
Selenium (Selenomax) . . . . 200 mcg
Green Tea Extract (standardized for 90%
   Catechins and 60% EGCG) . . . . 10 mg

NATURE'S HERBS®

600 East Quality Drive
American Fork, UT 84003

NATURE'S HERBS®
POWER-HERBS TOMATO-POWER

One (1) Softgel capsule provides:
LYC-O-MATO™ Natural Tomato Lycopene . . . . . 10 mg

BRONSON®

600 East Quality Drive
American Fork, UT 84003
Order direct 24 hours a day, 7 days a week
Tel: 1-800-235-3200 • Fax: 1-801-756-5739

BRONSON®
TOMATO-POWER

One (1) Softgel capsule provides:
LYC-O-MATO™ . . . . 10 mg

Tomato Power

References

Chapter 1   IN THE BEGINNING

1. Giovannucci, Edward et al., *"Intake of Carotenoids and Retinol in Relation to Risk of Prostate Cancer,"* *Journal of the National Cancer Institute,* 1995; 87: 1767-1776

2 Ibid., *"Carotenoids and Prostate Cancer, Follow-On Study,"* SDI Systems, Inc., March 17, 1997.

3.   Ibid.

4. Giovannucci, Edward et al, *"Intake of Carotenoids and Retinol in Relation to Risk of Prostate Cancer,"* Journal of the National Cancer Institute, 1995; 87: 1767-76.

5. Haney, Daniel Q., *"Tomatoes, Oranges, Pasta and Soybeans Studied as Cancer Fighters,"* Associated Press, April 14, 1997.

6. Erdman, John W., et al, *"Absorption and Transport of Carotenoids,"* from Carotenoids in Human Health, Vol. 69 of the Annals of the New York Academy of Sciences, Dec. 31, 1993, pp 76-77.

7. Tomato Research Council, News Story, *"Lycopene in the American Diet,"* Undated.

8. Giovannucci, Edward et al, *"Intake of Carotenoids and Retinol in Relation to Prostate Cancer,"* Journal of the National Cancer Institute 1985; 87: 1767-76.

9. Raloff, Janet, *"Radical Prostates: Female Hormones Now Play a Pivitol Role in a Distinctively Male Epidemic,"* Science News, February 22, 1997.

Chapter 2 SPECIAL PROTECTION FOR WOMEN

1. Haney, *Daniel Q., "Tomatoes, Oranges, Pasta and Soybeans Studied as Cancer Fighters,"* Associated Press, April 14, 1997

2. Kumpulainen, Jorma T. et al, *"Natural Antioxidants and Food Quality in Atherosclerosis and Cancer Prevention,"* Royal Society of Chemistry Information Services. (No date given.)

3. Levy, Joseph et al, *"The Tomato Carotenoid Lycopene and Cancer"* (Publication and date not given.)

4. Kobayshi, Takao et al, *"Effects of Lycopene, a Carotenoid on Intrathymic T Cell Differentiation and Peripheral CD4/CD9 Ratio in a High Mammary Tumor Strain on SHN Retired Mice,"* Anti-Cancer Drugs, Vol. 7, 1996.

5. Balch, James, *The Superantioxidants.* p 130.

6. Ernster, L. et al, *Experimental Cell Research,* 1959, 16, 7-14.

7. Ribaya-Mercado, J.. et al, *"Lycopene in Human Skin is Preferentially Consumed, Compared to Beta-Carotene, During Ultraviolet Irradiation,"* Agricultural Research Service. (Undated)

8. Rudinsky, M., et al, *"Protection by Lycopene in Lethal Radiation Exposure of Test Animals."* Radiasionnaia Biologica Radioecol, 1994. 34: 439-45.

Chapter 3 VERSATILE DEFENDER

1. Levy, Joseph, et al, *"Lycopene is a More Potent Inhibitor of Human Cancer Cell Proliferation Than Either a-Carotene or B-Carotene,"* Nutrition and Cancer," 1995: Vol, 24, No. 3; 257-266.

2. Goodman, M.T. et al, *"Dietary Factors in Lung Cancer Prognosis,"* European Journal Cancer (1992) 28:495-501.

3. *"Can Lycopene Contribute to Lower Lung Cancer?"* AP Worldstream, April 14, 1997.

4. Ibid.

5. Bohm, F. et al, *"Carotenoids Protect Against Cell Membranes Damaged by Nitrogen Dioxide Radicals,"* Letters to the Editor, Nature Medicine, Vol. 1, No. 2, February 1995, pp 98-99.

6. *"Can Lycopene Contribute to Lower Lung Cancer,"* AP Worldstream AP, April 14, 1997.

7. Franceschi, S. et al, *"Tomatoes and the Risk of Digestive Tract Cancers,"* International Journal Cancer, 1994, October 15, 59 (2):

8. Kamen, Betty, *"Lycopene: The Carotenoid King,"* Health Newsline, March, 1997.

9. Harman, Denham, Personal Communication, December 12, 1996.

10. Ames, Bruce N. et al, *"Oxidants, Antioxidants and Degenerative Diseases in Aging,"* Proceedings of the National Academy of Science, Vol, 90, September, 1993; 7915-7922.

11. Martin, Simon, *"Is This the Most Powerful Antioxidant Yet Found?"*

Chapter 4 INSURANCE FOR HEART, EYES AND BRAIN

1. Passwater, Richard A., Ph.D., Segment of The Nutrition Superbook: *"The Antioxidants "* (Edited by Jean Barilla); New Canaan, CT.: Keats Publishing, Inc., 1995.

2. Aviram, Michael, Ph.D., *"Lycopene and Atherosclerosis,"* A publication of Technion-Israel Institute of Technology. (Undated)

3. Lifetime Health Letter, University of Texas Houston Health Science Center, *"Heart Attack May Damage the Brain,"* May, 1994.

4. Personal Communication with Dr. Marion Diamond, Jan 1996.

5. *"Lycopene and Functional Capacity,"* Tomato Research Digest, Vol. 1, Fall 1996.

6. Boorsalis, Marie G. et al, *"Acute Phase Response and Plasma Carotenoid in Older Women: Findings in the Nun Study,"* Applied Nutritional Investigation, 1996; Vol. 12, Numbers 7/8: 475-78.

7. Meres-Perlman, Julie A., Ph.D., *"Serum Antioxidants and Age-Related Macular Degeneration in a Population-Based Case-Control Study,"* Archives Ophthalmology, December, 1995, Vol. 113: 1518-1523.

8. DiMascio, P. et al, *"Lycopene as the Most Efficient Biological Carotenoid Singlet Oxygen Quencher,"* Archives Biochemical Biophysics 1989; 274: 532-538.

Chapter 5 IMPORTANCE OF TESTING

1. Harman, Denham, Personal Communication, December 12, 1996.

2. Pryor, William A., Ph.D., Personal Communication, June 17, 1998. 3. Passwater, Richard A., Ph.D., Personal Communication, December 1996.

4. *"Life Extenders and Memory Boosters"* (Contributions by Life Extension Authorities, Reno, Nevada, Health Quest Publications, 1993, pp 33-35.

5. Thomas, Charles A., Jr., Personal Communication, June 15, 1998.

Chapter 6 BEHIND THE STORY

1. Nir, Zohar, Ph.D., Hartal, Dov, Ph.D., Raveh, Yigal, Ph.D., *"Lycopene From Tomatoes,"* International Food Ingredients, Issue 6, 1993, United Kingdom.

GLOSSARY

African-American Diet: Heavy on processed foods including white flour products, sugared cereals, some meats, and small amounts of vegetables and fruits, this diet uses tomatoes only infrequently.

Androgens: Male sex hormones that bring about male sexual characteristics and functions in men and help to maintain them.

Antioxidants: Substances such as lycopene, beta carotene and vitamins A, C, and E, as well as minerals such as selenium, protect our trillions of cells from oxidation, harm caused by oxygen. Oxygen is a must for us to convert foods to energy and warmth. (It is as necessary as oxygen used with gasoline for ignition by spark plugs to power our automobiles.) As a result of this oxidation, byproducts result: free radicals that harm our cells. Antixodants snuff out harmful free radicals.

Asian-American Diet: Rice is the staple food for Asian-Americans, as it is for Asians in their native countries. Whole grain rice with all its nutrients is growing in popularity in most of this population. Seafoods and sea vegetables are most popular. Tomatoes are rarely used in Oriental cooking.

Carcinogenic: Cancer-causing.

Carotenoids: Orange, red and yellow coloring substances in plants and animals are carotenoids. The word "carotenoid" originated from the fact that the first of such pigments were found in carrots. There are an estimated 600 carotenoids. Various authorities state that from eight to 12 are usable by the human body.

Degenerative Diseases: Ailments which involve a decline in structure and/or function. These include cancer, blockage of arteries, heart disease and diabetes.

Detoxification: As our lungs take in oxygen and circulating blood delivers it to our cells, a waste product is generated: carbon dioxide. This is sent to the lungs, which discharge it. All human processes are not 100 percent efficient. So some toxins (poisons) remain behind. The same goes for food taken in and discharged from the bowels as waste -- especially when bowel movement is not regular. Further, toxins in the environment -- the air we breathe, the food we eat and the water we drink -- bring us toxins we don't need. Detoxification is getting rid of these body poisons.

Enzymes: These protein-like substances in the human body bring about or speed up chemical changes in our cells from head to toe without themselves being changed. Enzymes are involved in all of our body processes, absorbing food, assimilating and using it. They make possible every body function from secreting and using hormones to the abilities to walk, think and remember.

Exudative Macular Degeneration: This is the wet form of macular degeneration, loss of function of the macula often leading to blindness, in which the cells give off (exude) moisture. There is also a dry form of macular degeneration.

Tomato Power

Free Radicals: Atoms or molecules with at least one unpaired electron are unstable and called free radicals. In order to become stable, they forcibly steal an electron from adjoining atoms or molecules. This act turns these atoms or molecules into free radicals. A chain reaction can start from this. Sufficient antioxidants are necessary to stop this process.

Genetic Engineering: Manipulating the DNA, the blueprint for cell replication, for the improvement of plants or animals is genetic engineering. It is feared by many individuals, because they feel insufficient research has been done in this field to guarantee that there will not be side effects from eating genetically engineered foods.

Holistic Medicine: A form of prevention or treatment of disease that accents dealing with all aspects of the individual -- body, mind, and/or spirit. Holistic medicine seeks to find and cope with basic causes for medical ailments, rather than symptoms, as with conventional medicine.

Lipoproteins: These are proteins combined with fats (lipids). Most well-known lipoproteins are low density lipoprotein (LDL), considered the harmful form of cholesterol, and high density lipoprotein (HDL), considered the helpful form of cholesterol.

Lymphocytes: White blood cells formed in the lymph glands, lymphocytes are important to the forming of antibodies, key soldiers in our immune system that defend us from harmful bacteria, viruses, cancer, and environmental toxins.

Macrophages: Large immune system cells in the lymph glands, liver and spleen. Their function is to work like PacMan, engulfing harmful bacteria, cellular debris, and foreign particles to keep us healthy.

Macular Degeneration: The word "macula" comes from the Latin, meaning a spot or stain. It is a small yellowish area in the center of the eye's retina, a light-sensitive membrane lining the inner eyeball and connected to the brain by the optic nerve. Macular degeneration is a major cause of blindness. It is brought about by blockage of blood circulation to the eyes, high blood pressure that may rupture micro-circulation, and damage caused by free radical attacks on the macula. (See free radicals in this glossary.)

Metabolism: This is a chemical and physical process that goes on inside our trillions of cells 24 hours a day. Nutrients combine with oxygen and thyroid hormone -- the regulator of metabolism -- to give our cells and us the energy to function and the heat to keep warm.

Metabolites: In the process of metabolism going on constantly in all of our trillions of cells, using nutrients, oxygen and thyroid hormone to develop energy and body warmth, byproducts are developed. These are called metabolites.

Mediterranean Diet: Italian foods including soups, salads, and pastas -- macaroni, ravioli, spaghetti -- and meat dishes usually contain tomatoes or tomato sauce. Tomato products, rich with the carotenoid lycopene, are thought to protect Italians and other European

Mediterranean populations from heart disease and cancer.

Mutagenic Agents: Substances or radiations, ultraviolet light or certain chemicals or drugs can cause changes (mutations) in cells. Some mutations are thought to open the way for normal cells to become abnormal or even cancerous.

Oxidation: See the definition of antioxidants above. Human life without oxidation of foods and their nutrients is not possible. However, oxidation causes free radicals -- also defined above -- making it necessary to have sufficient antioxidants to block the attacks on healthy cells. Antioxidants are made by the human body, and some come to us in foods and beverages. However, these are often insufficient, making it necessary to take antioxidant supplements such as lycopene and beta carotene, among others, to protect us from free radical attacks.

Parkinson's Disease: This is a progressive nervous system disease that occurs in the later years. Its major symptoms are nervous tremors, shaking palsy, partial facial paralysis, unstable walk and general weakness.

Proliferation: Growing or multiplying rapidly.

Prostate: This gland surrounds the urethra, the tube through which males discharge urine. With age, it becomes enlarged and tightens around the urethra, making the discharge of urine difficult, slow and often, intermittent. Called benign prostatic hypertrophy (BPH), this condition can lead to prostate cancer.

Replication: The process of duplicating and reproducing something, such as human cells.

Tocopherols: A group of four oils that make up the vitamin E complex. They occur mainly in wheat germ oil, sunflower seeds, sesame seeds, and hazelnuts.

INDEX

A

Absorption
  antioxidants from raw
    vegetables, 32
  lycopene absorption,
    encouragement by oils,
    23, 31, 81
African-American diet
  definition, 103
**Age-related macular
degeneration (ARMD)**
  causes, 68—69
  prevention
    lutein, 30—31
    lycopene, 30—31, 69—70
    vitamin C, 70
    vitamin E, 69—70
    zeaxanthin, 31
Aging
  antioxidant status, 76
  beta-carotene levels, 67
  lycopene levels, 67
Alpha-carotene
  cancer prevention, 30
  sources, 30
Androgen
  definition, 103
Antioxidant
  definition, 103
Antioxidant testing
  cost and reimbursement, 77
  frequency, 76
  importance, 61, 71—72
  Pantox panel, 74—79
  prescriptions, 72
  preventive medicine, 79
  specimen kit, 77
  supplementation
    recommendations, 76
ARMD, *see* Age-related
  macular degeneration
Asian-American diet
  definition, 103
Atherosclerosis
  cholesterol levels, 61, 73
  lycopene protection
    adipose tissue levels and
      myocardial infarction
      risk, 64
    low-density lipoprotein
      protection, 62
    LYC-O-MATO inhibition
      of plaques, 17
    overview, 15—16
    oxidation of low-density
      lipoprotein, 61—62
    vascular dementia
      association, 64—65
    vitamin E protection, 61

B

Beta-carotene
  absorption from raw
    vegetables, 32
  aging effects on levels, 67
  antioxidant activity, 30
  heating of foods and
    bioavailability, 32
  low-density lipoprotein
    protection against
    oxidation, 62
  lung cancer prevention,
    49—50
  lymphocyte protection
    from radiation, 51—52

popularity as supplement,
81—82
prostate cancer
prevention, 20—23, 26
sources, 30
structure, 28
synthesis for use as
supplements, 88
vitamin A processing, 27—29
Blood levels, lycopene
aging effects, 67
alcohol consumption
effects, 52
lung cancer, 50
prostate cancer, 40
serum levels in various
countries, 23—24
Brain cancer
gloma inhibition by
lycopenes, 43
Breast cancer
adipose tissue levels of
carotenoids, 46
lycopene prevention
comparison with other
carotenoids, 41—42, 44
inhibition in experimental
models, 43—45
mechanisms, 45
trends in incidence, 40—41
Bronson™ Laboratories
lycopene supplements, 93

C

Cancer, *see also* Breast cancer;
Brain cancer; Cervical intra-
epithelial neo-plasia;
Endometrial cancer; Lung
cancer; Prostate cancer; Skin
cancer

beta-carotene prevention
lung cancer, 49—50
prostate cancer, 20—23, 26
lycopene prevention
mechanisms, 33—35, 43,
45, 50—51, 58—59
overview, 15—16, 52
serum levels in cancer
patients, 40
Carbon tetrachloride
lycopene protection against
effects, 58
Carcinogenic
definition, 103
Carotenoids
adipose tissue levels in
breast cancer, 46
classification, 27
combination supplements,
84—85
definition, 103—104
prostate cancer prevention,
ranking by effectiveness,
20—23, 26
vitamin A processing, 27—29
**Cervical intra-epithelial
neoplasia (CIN)**
lycopene protection, 39—40
CIN,
see Cervical intra-epithelial
neoplasia
Cryptoxanthin
cancer prevention, 30
sources, 30

D

Degenerative disease
definition, 105

blood levels
  aging effects, 67
  alcohol consumption
    effects, 52
  lung cancer, 50
  prostate cancer, 40
  serum levels in various
    countries, 23—24
brain function protection,
  65—66
cancer prevention, *see also*
  Breast cancer; Brain
  cancer;
Cervical intra-epithelial
neoplasia; Endometrial
cancer; Lung cancer; Prostate
cancer; Skin cancer
  mechanisms, 33—35, 43,
    45, 50—51, 58—59
  overview, 15—16, 52
  serum levels in cancer
    patients, 40, 50
discovery, 82
enriched tomatoes,
  characteristics, 17—18, 83
immune cell protection,
  48, 51—52, 70
macular degeneration
  prevention, 30—31, 69—70
manufacturers of supple-
  ments, *see also* LYC-O-MATO
  Bronson^{TM} Laboratories,
    93
  Nature's Herb^{TM}, 92—93
  Twinlab^{TM}, 91—92
metabolites, 59
radiation, protection of
  effects, 46—48, 51—52, 82
sources
  other than tomato, 31—32

tomato food type and
  bioavailability, 32—33
structure, 28
tissue distribution, 16, 22
Lymphocyte
  antioxidant protection,
    48, 51—52, 70
  definition, 105

M

Macrophage
  definition, 106
Macular degeneration
  causes, 68—69
  definition, 106
  prevention
    lutein, 30—31
    lycopene, 30—31, 69—70
    vitamin C, 70
    vitamin E, 69—70
    zeaxanthin, 31
Mediterranean diet
  definition, 106—107
Memory
  antioxidant effects, 74
Metabolism
  definition, 106
Metabolites
  definition, 106
Mutagenic agent
  definition, 107
Myocardial infarction,
  see Atherosclerosis

N

Nature's Herb^{TM}
  lycopene supplements,
    92—93

PUBLICATIONS
(To Order Call 1-888-841-8007 *Except Where Noted)

The Cooking Cardiologist *(Video - 50 Minutes)* - Dr. Richard Collins, a cardiologist and leading researcher on reversing heart disease discusses and demonstrates how to cook delicious healthy meals that can lessen the risk of cardiovascular disease and improve one's overall health - 50 minute video. $19.95

The Cooking Cardiologist by Dr. Richard Collins - over 350 luscious recipes to lower cholesterol reduce the risk of heart disease, lower weight and improve health through the addition of plant proteins, fiber, and foods high in 3-omega fatty acids to your favorite recipes. Hard cover, 224 pages. $21.95

The Consumer's Guide To Herbal Medicine by Dr. Steven B. Karch, M.D. - a professional medical review of 65 of the most widely used herbs, their use, benefits and effectiveness; safety considerations, drug interactions, including German Government Commission E recommendations of which every user of herbs should be aware. Hard cover, 224 pages. $29.95

Tomato Power by James F. Scheer with Forward by James F. Balch, M.D. - discusses the benefits of a super-antioxidant, lycopene, that can slow aging and reduce heart disease and cancer risks. Soft cover, 116 pages. $12.95

Sex Pills A-Z, from Androstenedione to Zinc. *What Works and What doesn't!* by Dr. Carlon M. Colker, M.D. - examines a plethora of sex enhancing substances for added pleasure, better sex, longer sex, restoring sex drive, reversing sexual dysfunction and improving sexual powers. Soft cover, 140 pages. $14.95

Optimum Sports Nutrition, *Your Competitive Edge,* by Dr. Michael Colgan - a complete guide to the nutritional requirements of athletes. Soft cover, 562 pages. $24.95

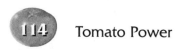

Muscular Development magazine - brings its readers the very best and latest scientific information on strength training, physique development, nutrition, health and fitness in an entertaining and contemporary format. 12 issues, ($2.50/copy - 50% off cover price). $29.94

Living Longer In The Boomer Age by Dr. John L. Zenk M.D. - discusses integrating alternative and conventional medicine. He describes the benefits of a new miracle anti-aging miracle supplement, 7-Keto DHEA for improving the immune system, losing fat and enhancing memory. *To order call 1-888-841-7996. $9.95

Periodization Breakthrough! *The Ultimate Training System* by Drs. Steven Fleck and William Kraemer. A straightforward explanation of periodized training. An essential system for successful strength training. Hard cover, 182 pages. *To order call 1-888-841-7996. $19.95

Muscle Meals by John Romano - a cookbook for bodybuilders and all athletes featuring a delicious array of easy-to-prepare energy-packed low-fat meals. Written by culinary expert, TV chef on ESPN's American Muscle Meals. Hard cover, 224 pages. *To order call 1-888-841-7996. $19.95

Mike Mentzer (New Advanced) High Intensity Training Program - a series of 4 audio-taped lectures, each approximately 50 minutes, by Mike Mentzer, Mr. Universe Champion, student and master of the art of bodybuilding. Included with these tapes is a 40-page High Intensity Training Program Guide; all attractively packaged. *To order call 1-888-841-7996. $39.95

INTERNET ORDERS

*These items can also be ordered via the internet
www.advancedresearchpress.com
click on the product mall to view.